Tea Tree Oil:
Improve Your Health
with the Amazing Benefits
of Tea Tree Oil

Contents

Introduction 1

Chapter 1 - Properties of Tea Tree Oil 3

    Properties of Tea Tree Oil 3

Chapter 2 - Skin and Hair Benefits 7

    Tea tree oil for acne 7

    Promotes hair growth 7

    Razor burn relief 7

    Dandruff cure 8

    Moisturizer 8

    Treatment for warts and corns 8

Chapter 3 - Tea Tree Oil Health Treatment 9

    Ear Infection 9

    Skin infections 9

    Toothaches 9

    Athlete's foot 10

    Cold sores 10

    Nail fungus 10

    Rashes 10

    Sore throat treatment 10

Head lice 11

Insect bites 11

Ringworm 11

Minor cuts 12

Arthritis 12

Chicken pox 12

Infected wounds...12

Strengthen immune system..........................12

Asthma 12

Chapter 4 - Beauty and Health Recipes.................14

Tea tree Oil Face Cleanser 14

Tea Tree Face Cream 15

Tea Tree Oil Honey Face Mask 16

Bug Bite Relief Stick 17

Cuticle softener 18

Tea Tree Oil Foot Soak 19

Whipped Vapor Rub 20

Tea Tree and Cucumber Balancing Lotion.........21

Antibacterial Hand Sanitizer 22

Tea Tree Foot Balm 23

Argan Oil and Tea Tree Moisturizing Stick 24

Rose Acne Face Mask 26

Oil Absorbing Face Cream for Oily Skin 27

Natural Antibacterial Toothpaste 28

Chapter 5 - Tea Tree Oil for Home Cleaner 29

Tea Tree and Lavender Surface Cleaner 29

Natural Liquid Dish Soap 30

Natural Air Freshener 30

Chapter 6 - How to Choose your Tea Tree Oil 31

Buy your Own Tea Tree Oil 31

Make Your Own Tea Tree Oil 32

Conclusion 34

Bonus Content! 36

Introduction

I want to thank you and congratulate you for downloading the book, *"Tea Tree Oil"*.

This book contains proven steps and strategies on how to use tea tree.

Tea tree oil or melaleuca oil is extracted from the leaves of tea tree. It should not be confused with camellia sinesis that is used to make tea. Tea tree plant is native to Australia. It is highly prized for its therapeutic and medicinal benefits. It was originally brewed or crushed and was used to treat infection and cuts.

Tea tree oil is known for its antifungal, antibacterial and antiviral properties. Many companies are now starting to recognize its benefit, so you can see it added to many commercial medicinal, beauty, bath and body products. Tea tree oil is a valuable component in your medicinal cabinet. It is very versatile since you can use it in different ways.

This book will show you how you can create basic antiseptic creams using tea tree oil. There are also recipes on homemade cleaners and body products.

This book will also provide you with tips on how to choose your own tea tree oil.

Thanks again for downloading this book, I hope you enjoy it!

Chapter 1 - Properties of Tea Tree Oil

Tea tree oil is extracted from the leaves of the tea tree which is also known as melaleuca alternifolia. It is found in the Southeast part of Australia. Despite what its name suggests, tea tree oil does not come from the tea plant used in making beverages. It is also different from tea oil, which is extracted from the tea plant.

Tea tree oil has many amazing benefits which is why it is popular all over the world. People use tea tree oil to cure almost all infections and diseases. It is usually found in most households in Australia especially those that have small children. Its healing and antibacterial properties can also boost your immunity. However, you must always remember to apply tea tree oil topically since it is poisonous when ingested.

Properties of Tea Tree Oil

Antibacterial

It is said that the best cures came from Mother Nature. There are many bacteria, fungi and viruses in nature so the plants have their own defense mechanism. Tea tree is a medicinal plant that contains potent antibacterial properties that can prevent and cure infection. You can apply tea tree oil topically to wounds to stop bacteria from spreading in the system.

Balsamic

Tea tree essential oil has balsamic properties that can improve your overall health. It can help improve the absorption of nutrients in the body and protect the system from disease as well.

Cicatristant

The Cricatristant in the oil is credited for its wound healing properties. It can also help reduce scarring from pox, acne, boils and wounds.

Antimicrobial

Tea tree oil has highly effective antimicrobial properties. The oils can prevent certain microbes from causing severe tropical fevers and malaria.

Antiviral

Viral infections are dangerous because they tend to reoccur. Virus can survive harsh conditions, so you cannot eliminate it simply by exposing it into high or low temperature because they develop a protective shell that shields them from it. Some viruses are even intelligent enough to develop a new protective mechanism every time they are activated in order to prevent the immune system from detecting them.

Viruses do not die naturally and can lie dormant for thousands of years. They only die by destroying their protective shell or by exposing them to very high temperature that are beyond their tolerance. Tea tree oil can rupture their protective barrier and can cure viral infections like pox, measles, mumps and even influenza.

Expectorant

Tea tree oil provides relief from cold, congestion and cough. You can rub it on the chest or inhale it.

Antiseptic

Open wounds are vulnerable to infections caused by fungi and bacteria that can lead to tetanus or sepsis. You can protect your wound with tea tree oil to prevent infection. It is just as effective as any antibiotic, but without any side effects.

Stimulant

Tea tree oil can stimulate hormone secretion and blood circulation. It can also boost the immune system to act as a shield from different types of infections. The reason why tea tree oil is popularly used in aromatherapy is that it can provide internal benefits without having to ingest the oil.

Sudorific

The accumulated toxins in the body also cause certain diseases. The toxins can be byproducts of a natural reaction or they can also enter the system through other ways. The body has a natural way to eliminate toxins including sweating or crying. Perspiration has many benefits since it can help remove toxins from the body and keep it cool.

Tea tree oil is a sudirific substance that can help remove toxins through sweat. It helps remove excess salt and water from the body while cleaning the pores as well.

Fungicide

Tea tree oil is also effective against fungal infections. It can stop the growth of fungus and treat conditions like Athlete's foot. Internal fungal infections are sometimes dangerous, but you should never ingest tea tree oil even after diluting it. There are other herbal remedies suited for internal infections.

A word of caution

There is no serious risk to applying tea tree oil on the skin, but in some rare cases, it may cause allergic reactions. Ingesting tea tree oil can have serious side effects including hallucinations, unsteadiness, rashes, weakness, blood cell abnormalities and confusion. Keep your tea tree oil away from pets and children.

Chapter 2 - Skin and Hair Benefits

Tea tree oil is often included in many beauty products because it has amazing skin and hair benefits.

Tea tree oil for acne

Tea tree oil is one of the best natural treatments for acne. Their natural antibacterial property is comparable to benzoyl peroxide. Unlike commercial acne treatments, it does not cause peeling or redness.

Simply apply the oil on the affected area using a Q-tip. Do not apply the oil all over the skin and only use it for spot treatment. Unclean makeup brushes can also cause acne. Make sure to wash your brushes regularly using shampoo and tea tree oil. You can also add the oil to a spray bottle and spray the brush in between uses to neutralize the bacteria.

Promotes hair growth

You can mix tea tree oil with other carrier oil and massage it in your scalp to help promote hair growth. Tea tree oil can unclog hair follicles and nourish the scalp. Always mix tea tree oil with a carrier oil because tea tree oil is too potent to use on its own.

Razor burn relief

Tea tree oil can sooth razor burns. You can mix it with coconut oil to help moisturize the skin at the same time.

Dandruff cure

Tea tree oil is also effective against dandruff. You can mix it to your shampoo and wash your scalp as usual.

Moisturizer

Tea tree oil combined with carrier oils is great for moisturizing dry skin. You can use it as a regular lotion or moisturizer. It is also effective especially on areas like the heels, knees and elbows.

Treatment for warts and corns

Warts are unpleasant to look at. Most treatments for warts include cauterization that involves burning the warts. Applying tea tree oil to the area is a natural and effective way to remove it. Apply the oil to the affected area twice a day. Be careful not to spill undiluted tea tree oil into other parts of the skin.

Chapter 3 - Tea Tree Oil Health Treatment

Tea tree oil is effective as a natural treatment for many conditions. You can use it as a first aid treatment before you try commercial drugs.

Ear Infection

Ear infections can be painful and uncomfortable. You can use tea tree as a natural treatment without getting the side effects of antibiotics. You simply rub 1-2 drops of the oil on the base of the ear every 3 hours to relieve the discomfort.

Skin infections

Tea tree oil is widely used for its antifungal and antibacterial benefits. It serves as a natural remedy for skin infections like ringworm. Dilute 5 drops of the oil in 1 tablespoon of coconut oil. The coconut oil also has its own antimicrobial properties so it is great to combine with tea tree oil. You can safely apply this in your skin 2-3 times in a day. However, avoid using this on genital area for yeast infection since it can sting badly.

Toothaches

Tea tree oil also works as an analgesic to numb tooth pain. You can dilute it with warm water and swish it in your mouth for a few minutes. To increase its potency, you can add one drop of clove oil. Be careful not to swallow the mixture.

Athlete's foot

Cure athlete's foot using tea tree oil. Combine 5 drops of the tea tree oil with 1 tablespoon of coconut oil and apply it to your feet. Massage it to clean skin and cover with socks before going to bed.

Cold sores

Combine 2 drops of tea tree oil with one teaspoon of carrier oil like olive or jojoba oil and apply to affected area twice or thrice a day.

Nail fungus

Natural treatment for nail fungus includes dietary changes and essential oils. Tea tree has antifungal properties that can kill nail fungus. Apply one drop of the oil on the affected area and rub to let it penetrate the area.

Rashes

There are many causes of rashes from food allergy to skin irritation. The best thing that you can do is to identify the cause of rashes to prevent any reoccurrence in the future. There are a lot of topical creams that can fade rashes. Try dabbing tea tree oil diluted with coconut oil every 3 hours until you see the rashes fade significantly.

Sore throat treatment

Sore throat is uncomfortable and inconvenient for anyone. Tea tree is a natural treatment for sore throat. Simply mix 3 drops of tea tree oil with boiling water. Drape a towel over your head and inhale the steam.

Inhale for about 5-8 minutes. This treatment is also effective in clearing chest and nose congestion. You can also mix the tea tree oil with water to make a gargle solution. Do this twice a day to kill bacteria in the tonsils and throat.

Head lice

Head lice are common in children, but anyone can get them. It usually spreads through head to head contact. The lice transfer from one person to another by crawling. Peppermint oil and tea tree extract can effectively repel head lice. Tea tree oil is also effective as a treatment for infected people. However, avoid using the oil in pets because it contains properties that are harsh for smaller animals.

Insect bites

Apply the tea tree oil to the area to prevent it from itching and to disinfect it. It is better if you cover it with a bandage to keep the oil from evaporating. Repeat the application twice or thrice a day.

Ringworm

Ringworm is a skin fungal infection that occurs when it is exposed to tinea. It is very contagious and can spread to other people or animal through contact. Use tea tree oil to prevent it from spreading. Apply the oil 3 times in a day. Make sure that you clean any item that may have come into contact with the fungus to prevent it from spreading further.

Minor cuts

Prevent infection by applying the tea tree oil on the affected area. Clean the cut well and apply the oil. You can cover it with a bandage.

Arthritis

Reduce the pain associated with arthritis by combining the tea tree oil with grape seed oil. Massage the mixture to the area twice or thrice a day. You can also use this to treat bruises.

Chicken pox

Chicken pox can leave unsightly marks on the skin. To prevent scarring, apply the tea tree oil directly to the blisters and let it dry. Dust it off with the corn starch. Repeat the process every 3 hours.

Infected wounds

Treat infected wounds by adding tea tree oil in a bowl of boiling water. Hold the affected area over the steam. You can also rinse the area with a combination of tea tree and water.

Strengthen immune system

Stimulate the immune system by diffusing in the air on a regular basis. You can also massage it on the soles of your feet to increase circulation and immune response.

Asthma

Tea tree oil can help relieve asthma and help you breathe easier. Pour two drops of carrier oil like jojoba or olive oil and 3 drops of tea tree oil in a pan that has been filled with water. Place the mixture over heat. As the mixture begins to boil, place a towel over your head and lean down to inhale the steam.

Chapter 4 - Beauty and Health Recipes

Using tea tree oil is easy and effective. Making your own beauty recipes is also more economical than commercial products.

Tea tree Oil Face Cleanser

½ cup grape seed oil

15 drop tea tree oil

¼ cup castor oil

¼ cup jojoba oil

Combine the oils in a large mixing bowl. Whisk the ingredients until combined. Pour the mixture in a clean jar. To use, dip clean fingers into the oil and massage it to your skin for 1-2 minutes until the oil is absorbed. Make sure to spread the oil into your neck. Dip your washcloth into hot water and place it over your face. This will allow your pores to open and remove any impurities. Wipe the oil from your face and pat dry with a towel. Use this method once a day. Increase the amount of jojoba oil if you have sensitive skin.

Tea Tree Face Cream

½ tbsp witch hazel extract

1 tbsp jojoba oil

¾ tsp stearic acid

40 drops tea tree oil

1 tbsp rosewater

½ tbsp hazelnut oil

2 tsp emulsifying wax

Combine the witch hazel and rosewater in a container. Mix the hazelnut oil and jojoba in another container. Add the wax and stearic acid in the third container. Place a pot over medium heat. Add water until it reaches about 3 inches. Simmer then add the wax mixture. Whisk the mixture until it becomes creamy white. This should take about 5 minutes. Add the remaining ingredients except for the tea tree oil.

Continue to whisk until the mixture is soft and light. Remove from the heat then add the tea tree oil. Whisk to cool the mixture until it starts to thicken on top. Transfer the mixture into a container with a lid. You can store this in the refrigerator for 30 days. Use the cream for acne prone skin.

Tea Tree Oil Honey Face Mask

1 tbsp honey

4 drops tea tree oil

Heat the honey in a small container. Stir in the tea tree oil. Apply to the whole face and wait for 20-25 minutes before rinsing it off. This face mask is effective in treating and preventing acne. Do this twice or thrice a week.

Bug Bite Relief Stick

1 tsp beeswax

3 tsp carnauba wax

2 ½ tsp calendula infused carrier oil

1 tsp vitamin E oil

1 ½ tsp castor oil

15 drops tea tree oil

10 drops lavender oil

3 drops peppermint oil

10 drops chamomile oil

5 drops vetiver oil

The beeswax and carnauba wax can harden the mixture so that it does not melt easily. This bug relief stick is great to take with you when you go outdoors. Most of the ingredients in this recipe have strong antiseptic, anti-inflammatory and insect repellant properties.

Fill a small pan with 2 cups of water then simmer. Add the carnauba wax and beeswax in a measuring cup. Place the measuring cup in the boiling water. Stir the mixture until it melts. Add the castor and calendula oil. Stir the mixture until it combines. Turn off the heat, but keep the cup in hot water. Add the essential oil and vitamin E oil. Stir gently. Transfer the mixture to a clean stick container. Let it solidify before using.

Cuticle softener

1 tbsp jojoba oil

10 drop tea tree oil

1 tbsp avocado oil

10 drop lavender oil

Tea tree oil is ideal to mix with other essential oils. The tea tree oil fights fungus while lavender oil promotes healing. Pour the avocado oil and jojoba oil in a dark bottle. Add the lavender and tea tree oil. Place the lid and shake the bottle to combine the ingredients. The dark bottle will help preserve the oils. To use, massage a few drops into your cuticles to soften it.

Tea Tree Oil Foot Soak

1 tbsp dried rosemary

1 tbsp fresh ginger, grated

1 tbsp baking soda

10 drops tea tree oil

1 tbsp dried sage

4 cups water

1 tbsp Epsom salt

Ice cubes

Place the ginger, rosemary and sage in a pan. Add the water and place over medium heat. Let it boil then remove from heat. Cover and set aside for 10 minutes. Add the tea tree oil and Epsom salt. Stir the mixture. Pour in a wide basin. Soak your feet and add more water if desired. Soak for 15 minutes then dry with towel.

Whipped Vapor Rub

¼ cup coconut oil

25 drops eucalyptus oil

15 drops lavender oil

10 drop tea tree oil

¼ cup Shea butter

20 drops peppermint oil

10 drop lemon oil

Whip the coconut oil in a bowl for a minute. Add the essential oils then stir it again using a clean spatula. Whip until the mixture is light and fluffy. Scoop the mixture into a jar. Make sure to store this in a cool and dry place. Use clean utensils with each use to prevent contamination. This natural vapor rub does not have the same immediate effect as commercial vapor rub. It seeps into the skin slowly and have a mild cooling effect. Apply the cream in your chest and back. You can also apply it in your hands and inhale the scent.

Tea Tree and Cucumber Balancing Lotion

20 g witch hazel

6 g jojoba seed oil

1 g liquid lecithin

2 g stearic acid

10 drop tea tree oil

20 g cucumber hydrosol

5 g hazelnut oil

4 g emulsifying wax

1 g vitamin E oil

2 g leucidal liquid

Pour the witch hazel and cucumber hydrosol in a cup. Set it in a double broiler. Measure the stearic acid, jojoba oil, liquid lecithin, hazelnut oil and emulsifying wax in a cup. Let it sit in a pot of simmering water. Remove from heat once it reaches 150 degrees. Pour the oil in a mixing bowl and whisk at medium speed. Add the cooled witch hazel mixture. Stir for 5 minutes. Add the tea tree oil, vitamin E and leucidal liquid into the mixture. Whisk the mixture until it is light. Pour in a container.

Antibacterial Hand Sanitizer

80 drops clover bud oil

40 drops cinnamon bark oil

30 drops tea tree oil

70 drops essential oil

30 drops eucalyptus oil

20 drops rosemary oil

Combine the ingredients in a dark bottle. Do not use this undiluted. You can use 10 drops of the mixture with every 120 grams of alcohol. Feel free to use vodka or even rubbing alcohol if you want.

Tea Tree Foot Balm

40 g Shea butter

20 g calendula oil

10 g jojoba oil

20 g sunflower oil

15 g beeswax

10 g or 100 drops tea tree oil

Measure the Shea butter in a glass cup. Set it in a pot of simmering water. Heat the butter for 20 minutes until it liquefies. Add the calendula oil and sunflower oil. Mix in the beeswax and jojoba oil. Let the beeswax melt for 10 minutes. Stir the ingredients until well combined. Add the tea tree oil and stir again. Pour the mixture in a 4-ounce container. Let it solidify before using.

Argan Oil and Tea Tree Moisturizing Stick

25 g argan oil

12 g beeswax

7 g soy wax

5 g shea butter

3 g vitamin E oil

1.5 ml rosemary extract

15 drops lemon oil

15 g evening primrose oil

10 g cocoa butter

5 g mango butter

3 g wheat germ oil

30 drops tea tree oil

Fill a Dutch oven with 4 cups of water then let it simmer. Add the beeswax and soy wax in the measuring cup. Stir the mixture until it melts. Combine the mango butter, Shea butter and cocoa butter in another measuring cup then place into the water bath until the mixture melts. Add vitamin E oil, Argan oil, wheat germ oil, evening primrose oil, rosemary extract and essential oil in a separate cup. Let the wax melt then add the argan oil to the mixture. Turn off the heat, but leave the cups in the water. Quickly pour the wax mixture into the water. Stir to combine. Add the wax and butter mixture to the argan oil. The mixture will start to harden so continue to mix until it melts again. Pour the mixture into a clean stick container and let it cool until it solidifies. Use as a portable moisturizer.

Rose Acne Face Mask

25 g fuller Earth clay

Small egg yolk

3 g Neem oil

1.5 ml tea tree oil

15 g aloe vera gel

6 g manuka honey

3 g fresh garlic clove

10 drops rose oil

Combine all of the ingredients in a food processor and blend until it is smooth and creamy. Apply the mixture all over your face. Leave for 15 minutes then rinse it off with warm water.

Oil Absorbing Face Cream for Oily Skin

20 g calendula hydrosol

17 g jojoba oil

2 g stearic acid

20 drops grapefruit seed extract

10 drops tea tree oil

10 g calendula extract

6 g emulsifying wax

2.5 g kaolin clay

10 drops lavender oil

3 drops grapefruit essential oil

Measure the hydrosol and pour it in a cup. Combine the emulsifying wax, kaolin clay, jojoba oil and stearic acid in another cup. Place the cups in a water bath. Heat the water until it reaches 140 degrees. Remove the cups from heat. Pour the liquid into a large bowl and whisk using a stick blender for 5 minutes. Add the grapefruit extract and other essential oils. Continue to whisk for 10 minutes until the cream starts to solidify. Transfer it into your container and keep refrigerated.

Natural Antibacterial Toothpaste

5 tbsp baking soda

6 drops tea tree oil

4 tbsp coconut oil

1 tsp ground sage

Combine all of the ingredients in a bowl until you have a smooth consistency. Scoop the mixture into your brush then store the remaining in a container. Use just like normal toothpaste.

Chapter 5 - Tea Tree Oil for Home Cleaner

Commercial home cleansers are full of chemicals and toxins that are harmful for your health. Fortunately, natural ingredients are also effective in removing dirt and grime. If you like the bubbles and foams that come from commercial cleansers, then it might take some time before you get used to homemade alternatives. However, these products are just as effective and are safer for you to use.

Tea Tree and Lavender Surface Cleaner

1 cup water

10 drops tea tree oil

¼ cup white vinegar

10 drops lavender oil

Mix the water and vinegar in your spray bottle. Add the tea tree oil. Replace the lid then shake the bottle to mix the ingredients. This recipe is a great all around cleanser. Simply spray on a surface and wipe with a towel.

Natural Liquid Dish Soap

1 ¾ cups water

1 tbsp bar soap, grated

1 tbsp baking soda

15 drops tea tree oil

Pour the water in a pot and let it boil. Mix the grated soap bar and baking soda in a bowl. Pour hot water in the bowl. Stir the mixture until it completely melts. Let it cool for 8 hours. Stir the mixture occasionally. Pour in a squirt bottle then add the tea tree oil. Shake the container before each use.

Natural Air Freshener

3 cloves

1 tbsp vodka

5 tbsp water

5 drops tea tree oil

Combine all of the ingredients in a spray bottle. Shake before using. This air freshener is effective, cheap and easy to make. It works great in eliminating bathroom and basement odor.

Chapter 6 - How to Choose your Tea Tree Oil

The chemicals in tea tree oil have many benefits. It is very versatile and is extremely useful in making beauty products and home cleaning products. Just like any product in the market, you also have to make sure that you are buying authentic tea tree oil. Here are some tips that can help you buy or make your own.

Buy your Own Tea Tree Oil

Determine the % of Terpinen 4 OL

All tea tree oil contains terpinen 4 OL, an active ingredient that serves as the primary antiseptic agent. The higher the percentage, the stronger the antiseptic property of the oil is. Tea tree oil sold in the market range from 10-40%. If you have sensitive skin, opt for a lower concentration, but if you are going to use the oil mainly for household cleaning, then you can opt for higher concentration.

Dark bottle

Studies show that terpinene 4 OL rapidly loses its potency when exposed to light. Light exposure can also increase para-cymene in the oil that triggers skin irritations.

Organic

You can choose to purchase certified organic tea tree oil depending on your needs. Certified organic products have better quality and concentration.

How much should it cost?

The total price of the tea tree oil depends based on the size and amount that you are buying, as well as the concentration of the oil. Large 32-ounce bottles can cost over $100 while 60 ml bottles can range from 10-20$.

Make Your Own Tea Tree Oil

You can also make your own tea tree oil if you are lucky enough to live in an area where tea tree naturally grows. Knowing how to make your own tea tree oil is beneficial during emergency situations.

Instructions:

1. Place the tea tree leaves in a pot. Pour enough water to submerge the leaves.
2. Place a steamer in the pot over the leaves and water.
3. Place a small heatproof cup inside the steamer.
4. Place the lid of the pot upside down. The handle should be inside the measuring cup.
5. Turn the heat high and let the water boil. The water should start to evaporate and condense. The vapor will be trapped in the lid and will flow into the measuring cup.
6. Place ice cubes on top of the lid to hasten the steaming process.

7. Turn off the heat once the ice melts.
8. Remove the lid and take the cup. Remember to use pot holders since the cup can be very hot.
9. Pour the contents of the cup into a separating funnel.
10. Make sure that the stopcock on the bottom is close. Invert the funnel and release the pressure. The oil will float on top.
11. Pour the tea tree oil in a separate container. Make sure to store your oil in a dark glass bottle.

Conclusion

As we learnt from this book some of the truly amazing properties of Tea Tree Oil that makes it a very popular natural agent in our modern day world for curing infectious organisms such as fungus, bacteria, and viruses. More importantly, it is also known to effectively fight a number of infections that are resistant to some antibiotics. Therefore, tea tree oil as we know is also an excellent natural remedy for hundreds of bacterial and fungal skin ailments such as acne, abscess, oily skin, blisters, sun burns, athlete's foot, warts, herpes, insect bites, rashes, dandruff and other minor wounds and irritations. A small bottle of tea tree oil can be inexpensively purchased from most supermarkets and pharmacists and should form part of your everyday home and or travelling medical kit.

Thank you again for downloading this book!

I hope this book was able to help you understand the amazing benefits of tea tree oil.

The next step is to use the oil for yourself.

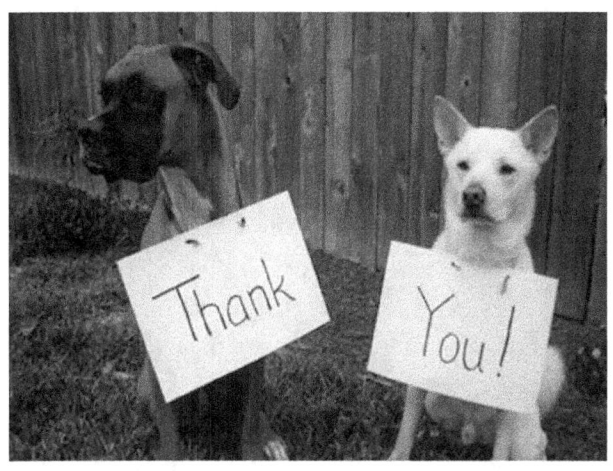

Finally, if you enjoyed this book, then I'd like to ask you for a favor, would you be kind enough to leave a review for this book on Amazon? It'd be greatly appreciated!

Thank you and good luck!

Bonus Content!

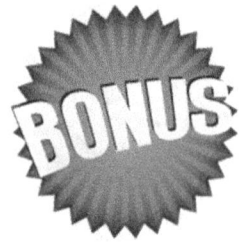

As a token of our appreciation <u>Grand Reveur Publications</u> would like to give you access to our exclusive bonus content (including free eBooks!).

<u>You're only a click away from receiving:</u>

Exclusive pre-release access to our latest eBooks

Free Grand Reveur eBooks during promotional periods

A method ANYONE can use to publish their own book and make passive income

https://ignorelimits.leadpages.net/grandreveurpublications/

As this is a limited time offer it would be a shame to miss out, I recommend grabbing these bonuses before reading on.

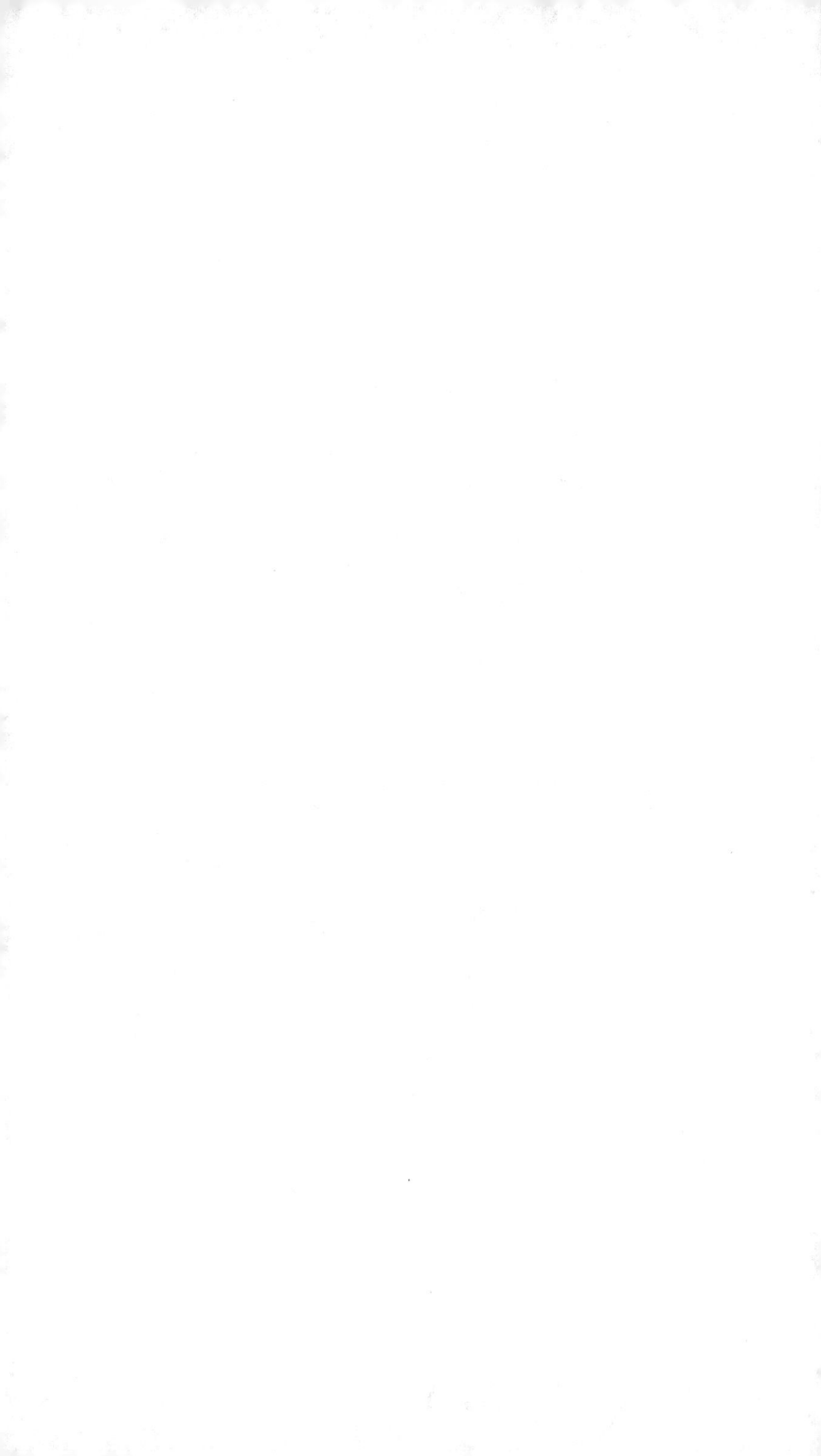